Competency Based Logbook in AETCOM, Medical Humanities, Sports and Extracurricular Activities

2

W0112662

Logbook for all Professional Years of MBBS

Compiled and structured as per the latest CBME Guidelines | Competency Based Undergraduate Curriculum for the Indian Medical Graduate

Name: _____

Roll No.: _____ University Registration No.: _____

Date of Admission: _____

Permanent Address: _____

E-mail ID: _____ Batch: _____

Mobile No.: _____

2

Competency Based Logbook in
AETCOM, Medical Humanities, Sports and Extracurricular Activities

Logbook for all Professional Years of MBBS

Compiled and structured as per the latest CBME Guidelines | Competency Based
Undergraduate Curriculum for the Indian Medical Graduate

Niket Verma MBBS, MD

Assistant Professor
Department of General Medicine
Army College of Medical Sciences
Delhi Cantt, New Delhi

Poonam Agrawal MBBS, MD (Biochemistry)

Professor and Head
Department of Biochemistry
Dr Baba Saheb Ambedkar Medical College and Hospital
New Delhi

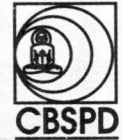

CBSPD

CBS Publishers & Distributors Pvt Ltd
New Delhi • Bengaluru • Chennai • Kochi • Kolkata • Lucknow • Mumbai
Hyderabad • Jharkhand • Nagpur • Patna • Pune • Uttarakhand

Disclaimer
Science and technology are constantly changing fields. New research and experience broaden the scope of information and knowledge. The authors have tried their best in giving information available to them while preparing the material for this book. Although all efforts have been made to ensure optimum accuracy of the material, yet it is quite possible some errors might have been left uncorrected. The publisher, the printer, and the authors will not be held responsible for any inadvertent errors or inaccuracies.

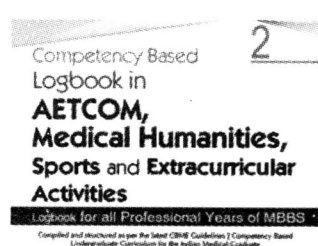

Competency Based
Logbook in
AETCOM,
Medical Humanities,
Sports and **Extracurricular**
Activities
Logbook for all Professional Years of MBBS
Compiled and structured as per the latest CBME Guidelines | Competency Based
Undergraduate Curriculum for the Indian Medical Graduate

ISBN: 978-93-89565-89-8

Copyright © Authors and Publisher

First Edition: 2021

Reprint: 2024

All rights are reserved. No part of this book may be reproduced or transmitted in any form or by any means, electronic or mechanical, including photocopying, recording, or any information storage and retrieval system without permission, in writing, from the authors and the publisher.

Published by **Satish Kumar Jain** and produced by **Varun Jain** for

CBS Publishers & Distributors Pvt Ltd

4819/XI Prahlad Street, 24 Ansari Road, Daryaganj, New Delhi 110 002, India
Ph: 011-23289259, 23266861   Website: www.cbspd.com
                                    e-mail: delhi@cbspd.com
Corporate Office: 204 FIE, Industrial Area, Patparganj, Delhi 110 092, India
Ph: 011-4934 4934   Fax: 011-4934 4935   e-mail: publishing@cbspd.com; publicity@cbspd.com

Branches

• **Bengaluru:** Seema House 2975, 17th Cross, K.R. Road, Banasankari 2nd Stage, Bengaluru 560 070, Karnataka, India
  Ph: +91-80-26771678/79   Fax: +91-80-26771680   e-mail: bangalore@cbspd.com
• **Chennai:** 7, Subbaraya Street, Shenoy Nagar, Chennai 600 030, Tamil Nadu, India
  Ph: +91-44-26680620, 26681266   Fax: +91-44-42032115   e-mail: chennai@cbspd.com
• **Kochi:** 42/1325, 1326, Power House Road, Opposite KSEB, Power House, Ernakulum 682018, Kochi, Kerala, India
  Ph: +91-484-4059061–65, 67   Fax: +91-484-4059065   e-mail: kochi@cbspd.com
• **Kolkata:** 147, Hind Ceramics Compound, 1st Floor, Nilgunj Road, Belghoria, Kolkata 700056, West Bengal, India
  Ph: +91-33-25633055/56   e-mail: kolkata@cbspd.com
• **Lucknow:** Basement, Khushnuma Complex, 7 Meerabai Marg (behind Jawahar Bhawan), Lucknow 226001, UP, India
  Ph: +91-522-4000032   e-mail: tiwari.lucknow@cbspd.com
• **Mumbai:** PWD Shed, Gala No. 25/26, Ramchandra Bhatt Marg, Next to JJ Hospital, Gate No. 2, Opp. Union Bank of India, Noorbaug
  Mumbai 400009, Maharashtra, India
  Ph: +91-22-66661880/89   e-mail: mumbai@cbspd.com

Representatives

• **Hyderabad**   0-9885175004   • **Jharkhand**   0-9811541605   • **Nagpur**   0-8692091830
• **Patna**   0-9334159340   • **Pune**   0-9664372571   • **Uttarakhand** 0-9716462459

Printed at: Mudrak, Noida, UP, India

Preface

The current Logbook encompasses **AETCOM, Medical Humanities, Sports and Extracurricular Activities.** This logbook has been designed keeping in mind the requirements of the new Competency Based Medical Education (CBME) Curriculum and is supposed to be maintained across all the professional years of MBBS.

The **AETCOM Module** has been incorporated as a longitudinal programme under the new curriculum where **34, 37, 25** and **43** hours have been allocated to AETCOM in the **First, Second, Third Part I** and **Third Part II Professional Years,** respectively. Correspondingly, the section on AETCOM in this logbook is divided across all four professional years. The 40 hours of AETCOM covered in the Foundation Course need to be recorded in a separate logbook *Logbook for Foundation Course for MBBS Students.*

The list of competencies to be included in each professional year and maximum number of attempts allowed for each activity is based on discretion of individual departments in collaboration with college medical education units. Adequate space is provided to enter the details of the competencies and activities, the details of remedial training (if any), the rating for each attempt at the activity and the final decision of the faculty. The assessment scale has only two ratings, 'Scope for further improvement' and 'Satisfactory'; thereby emphasising on positive motivation for all students.

While the new curriculum includes **Medical Humanities** only under the components of First Professional MBBS, we have incorporated Medical Humanities in all four professional years in this logbook as this topic is closely interlinked with professional development and AETCOM.

A total of 60 and 28 hours have been allocated to **Sports and Extracurricular Activities** in First and Second Professional MBBS respectively under the new curriculum. This section is correspondingly divided across the first two professional years. The 22 hours allocated to Sports and Extracurricular Activities under the foundation course need to be recorded in a separate logbook *Logbook for Foundation Course for MBBS Students.*

The sections on medical humanities and sports and extracurricular activities are designed as **Reflective Portfolios** with space for reflection writing by the learners. Separate pages are provided for recording the details of any assignments and assessments on these topics.

Niket Verma
drniketacme@gmail.com

Poonam Agrawal
drpoonam24agrawal@yahoo.com

Certificate A1

It is hereby certified that Ms./Mr. ...., Roll No./University Registration No. ...., who is a student of MBBS at ....…................................... (name of Medical College), has satisfactorily achieved the competencies and completed the assignments relevant for Ist Professional MBBS.

She/He is eligible to appear for the Ist Professional MBBS University examinations which will be conducted by .... (name of the affiliating university), from .... to ....

Signature of Faculty-in-charge

Signature of Head of the Department

Signature of Principal/Dean of the College

Certificate B1

It is hereby certified that Ms./Mr. ...., Roll No./University Registration No. ...., who is a student of MBBS at ….....…..............................…...............……. (name of Medical College), has NOT achieved the competencies and/or completed the assignments relevant for Ist Professional MBBS.

She/He is NOT eligible to appear for the Ist Professional MBBS University examinations which will be conducted by .... (name of the affiliating university), from .... to ....

Signature of Faculty-in-charge

Signature of Head of the Department

Signature of Principal/Dean of the College

Certificate A2

It is hereby certified that Ms./Mr. ....,
Roll No./University Registration No. ...., who is a student of MBBS
at ....(name of Medical College), has satisfactorily achieved the competencies
and completed the assignments relevant for IInd Professional MBBS.

She/He is eligible to appear for the IInd Professional MBBS University examinations which will be conducted
by .... (name of the affiliating university), from .... to ....

Signature of Faculty-in-charge

Signature of Head of the Department

Signature of Principal/Dean of the College

Certificate B2

It is hereby certified that Ms./Mr. ....,
Roll No./University Registration No. ...., who is a student of MBBS
at ....…….. (name of Medical College), has NOT achieved the competencies
and/or completed the assignments relevant for IInd Professional MBBS.

She/He is NOT eligible to appear for the IInd Professional MBBS University examinations which will be conducted
by .... (name of the affiliating university), from .... to ....

Signature of Faculty-in-charge

Signature of Head of the Department

Signature of Principal/Dean of the College

Certificate A3

It is hereby certified that Ms./Mr. ....,
Roll No./University Registration No. ...., who is a student of MBBS
at ....…….. (name of Medical College), has satisfactorily achieved the competencies
and completed the assignments relevant for IIIrd Professional MBBS (Part I).

She/He is eligible to appear for the IIIrd Professional MBBS (Part I) University examinations which will be
conducted by .... (name of the affiliating university), from .... to ....

Signature of Faculty-in-charge

Signature of Head of the Department

Signature of Principal/Dean of the College

Certificate B3

It is hereby certified that Ms./Mr. ....,
Roll No./University Registration No. ...., who is a student of MBBS
at . ...……. (name of Medical College), has NOT achieved the competencies
and/or completed the assignments relevant for IIIrd Professional MBBS (Part I).

She/He is NOT eligible to appear for the IIIrd Professional MBBS (Part I) University examinations which will be
conducted by .... (name of the affiliating university), from .... to ....

Signature of Faculty-in-charge

Signature of Head of the Department

Signature of Principal/Dean of the College

Certificate A4

It is hereby certified that Ms./Mr. ....,
Roll No./University Registration No. ...., who is a student of MBBS
at .... (name of Medical College), has satisfactorily achieved the competencies
and completed the assignments relevant for IIIrd Professional MBBS (Part II).

   She/He is eligible to appear for the IIIrd Professional MBBS (Part II) University examinations which will be
conducted by .... (name of the affiliating university), from .... to ....

Signature of Faculty-in-charge

Signature of Head of the Department

Signature of Principal/Dean of the College

Certificate B4

It is hereby certified that Ms./Mr. ....,
Roll No./University Registration No. ...., who is a student of MBBS
at .... (name of Medical College), has NOT achieved the competencies
and/or completed the assignments relevant for IIIrd Professional MBBS (Part II).

   She/He is NOT eligible to appear for the IIIrd Professional MBBS (Part II) University examinations which will
conducted by .... (name of the affiliating university), from .... to ....

Signature of Faculty-in-charge

Signature of Head of the Department

Signature of Principal/Dean of the College

Contents

Preface   *v*

---

1. **Attitude, Ethics and Communication (AETCOM)**

   A. Ist Professional MBBS   3

   B. IInd Professional MBBS   17

   C. IIIrd Professional MBBS (Part I)   31

   D. IIIrd Professional MBBS (Part II)   45

2. **Medical Humanities**

   A. Ist Professional MBBS   61

   B. IInd Professional MBBS   72

   C. IIIrd Professional MBBS (Part I)   77

   D. IIIrd Professional MBBS (Part II)   82

3. **Sports and Extracurricular Activities**

   A. Ist Professional MBBS   89

   B. IInd Professional MBBS   108

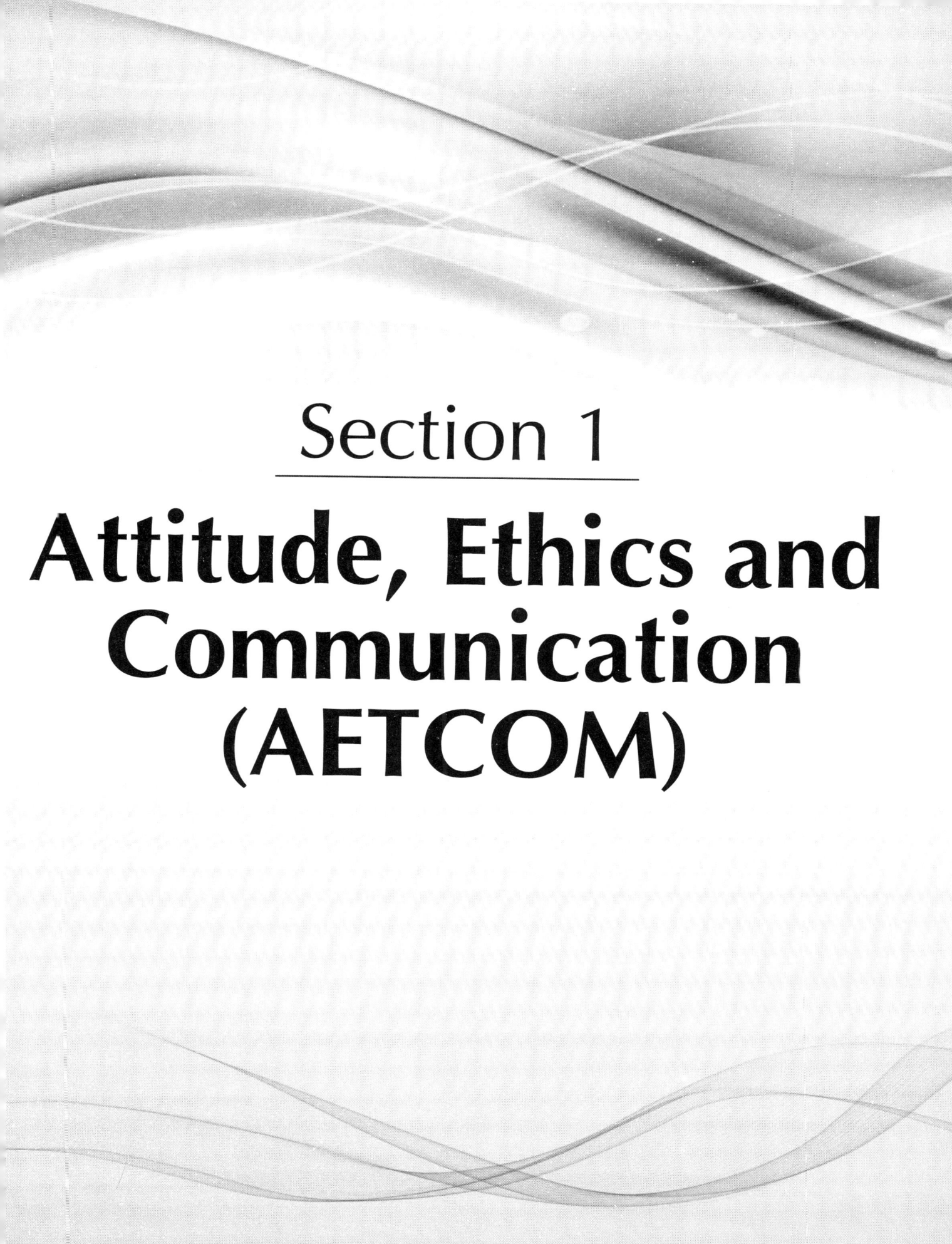

Section 1

Attitude, Ethics and Communication (AETCOM)

A. Ist Professional MBBS

Sr. No.	Competency number and description of the activity	Maximum number of attempts allowed for the activity	No. of attempts taken by the learner (with date of each attempt)	Any remedial training needed? (Yes / No) If yes then state the reason(s)	Rating 1. Scope for further improvement 2. Satisfactory (All attempts at the activity must be rated separately)	Final decision of faculty C—Completed N—Not completed	Feedback conveyed by faculty (Yes / No) Signature of faculty (with date)	Feedback received by learner (Yes / No) Signature of learner (with date)
1.								
2.								
3.								
4.								
5.								

A. Ist Professional MBBS

Sr. No.	Competency number and description of the activity	Maximum number of attempts allowed for the activity	No. of attempts taken by the learner (with date of each attempt)	Any remedial training needed? (Yes / No) If yes then state the reason(s)	Rating 1. Scope for further improvement 2. Satisfactory (All attempts at the activity must be rated separately)	Final decision of faculty C—Completed N—Not completed	Feedback conveyed by faculty (Yes / No) Signature of faculty (with date)	Feedback received by learner (Yes / No) Signature of learner (with date)
6.								
7.								
8.								
9.								
10.								

A. Ist Professional MBBS

Sr. No.	Competency number and description of the activity	Maximum number of attempts allowed for the activity	No. of attempts taken by the learner (with date of each attempt)	Any remedial training needed? (Yes / No) If yes then state the reason(s)	Rating 1. Scope for further improvement 2. Satisfactory (All attempts at the activity must be rated separately)	Final decision of faculty C—Completed N—Not completed	Feedback conveyed by faculty (Yes / No) Signature of faculty (with date)	Feedback received by learner (Yes / No) Signature of learner (with date)
11.								
12.								
13.								
14.								
15.								

A. Ist Professional MBBS

Sr. No.	Competency number and description of the activity	Maximum number of attempts allowed for the activity	No. of attempts taken by the learner (with date of each attempt)	Any remedial training needed? (Yes / No) If yes then state the reason(s)	Rating 1. Scope for further improvement 2. Satisfactory (All attempts at the activity must be rated separately)	Final decision of faculty C—Completed N—Not completed	Feedback conveyed by faculty (Yes / No) Signature of faculty (with date)	Feedback received by learner (Yes / No) Signature of learner (with date)
16.								
17.								
18.								
19.								
20.								

A. Ist Professional MBBS

Sr. No	Competency number and description of the activity	Maximum number of attempts allowed for the activity	No. of attempts taken by the learner (with date of each attempt)	Any remedial training needed? (Yes / No) If yes then state the reason(s)	Rating 1. Scope for further improvement 2. Satisfactory (All attempts at the activity must be rated separately)	Final decision of faculty C—Completed N—Not completed	Feedback conveyed by faculty (Yes / No) Signature of faculty (with date)	Feedback received by learner (Yes / No) Signature of learner (with date)
21.								
22.								
23.								
24.								
25.								

A. Ist Professional MBBS

Sr. No.	Competency number and description of the activity	Maximum number of attempts allowed for the activity	No. of attempts taken by the learner (with date of each attempt)	Any remedial training needed? (Yes / No) If yes then state the reason(s)	Rating 1. Scope for further improvement 2. Satisfactory (All attempts at the activity must be rated separately)	Final decision of faculty C—Completed N—Not completed	Feedback conveyed by faculty (Yes / No) Signature of faculty (with date)	Feedback received by learner (Yes / No) Signature of learner (with date)
26.								
27.								
28.								
29.								
30.								

A. Ist Professional MBBS

Sr. No.	Competency number and description of the activity	Maximum number of attempts allowed for the activity	No. of attempts taken by the learner (with date of each attempt)	Any remedial training needed? (Yes / No) If yes then state the reason(s)	Rating 1. Scope for further improvement 2. Satisfactory (All attempts at the activity must be rated separately)	Final decision of faculty C—Completed N—Not completed	Feedback conveyed by faculty (Yes / No) Signature of faculty (with date)	Feedback received by learner (Yes / No) Signature of learner (with date)
31.								
32.								
33.								
34.								
35.								

A. Ist Professional MBBS

Sr. No.	Competency number and description of the activity	Maximum number of attempts allowed for the activity	No. of attempts taken by the learner (with date of each attempt)	Any remedial training needed? (Yes / No) If yes then state the reason(s)	Rating 1. Scope for further improvement 2. Satisfactory (All attempts at the activity must be rated separately)	Final decision of faculty C—Completed N—Not completed	Feedback conveyed by faculty (Yes / No) Signature of faculty (with date)	Feedback received by learner (Yes / No) Signature of learner (with date)
36.								
37.								
38.								
39.								
40.								

A. Ist Professional MBBS

Sr. No	Competency number and description of the activity	Maximum number of attempts allowed for the activity	No. of attempts taken by the learner (with date of each attempt)	Any remedial training needed? (Yes / No) If yes then state the reason(s)	Rating 1. Scope for further improvement 2. Satisfactory (All attempts at the activity must be rated separately)	Final decision of faculty C—Completed N—Not completed	Feedback conveyed by faculty (Yes / No) Signature of faculty (with date)	Feedback received by learner (Yes / No) Signature of learner (with date)
41.								
42.								
43.								
44.								
45.								

A. Ist Professional MBBS

Sr. No.	Competency number and description of the activity	Maximum number of attempts allowed for the activity	No. of attempts taken by the learner (with date of each attempt)	Any remedial training needed? (Yes / No) If yes then state the reason(s)	Rating 1. Scope for further improvement 2. Satisfactory (All attempts at the activity must be rated separately)	Final decision of faculty C—Completed N—Not completed	Feedback conveyed by faculty (Yes / No) Signature of faculty (with date)	Feedback received by learner (Yes / No) Signature of learner (with date)
46.								
47.								
48.								
49.								
50.								

A. Ist Professional MBBS

Sr. No.	Competency number and description of the activity	Maximum number of attempts allowed for the activity	No. of attempts taken by the learner (with date of each attempt)	Any remedial training needed? (Yes / No) If yes then state the reason(s)	Rating 1. Scope for further improvement 2. Satisfactory (All attempts at the activity must be rated separately)	Final decision of faculty C—Completed N—Not completed	Feedback conveyed by faculty (Yes / No) Signature of faculty (with date)	Feedback received by learner (Yes / No) Signature of learner (with date)
51.								
52.								
53								
54.								
55.								

A. Ist Professional MBBS

Sr. No.	Competency number and description of the activity	Maximum number of attempts allowed for the activity	No. of attempts taken by the learner (with date of each attempt)	Any remedial training needed? (Yes / No) If yes then state the reason(s)	Rating 1. Scope for further improvement 2. Satisfactory (All attempts at the activity must be rated separately)	Final decision of faculty C—Completed N—Not completed	Feedback conveyed by faculty (Yes / No) Signature of faculty (with date)	Feedback received by learner (Yes / No) Signature of learner (with date)
56.								
57.								
58.								
59.								
60.								

A. Ist Professional MBBS

Sr. No.	Competency number and description of the activity	Maximum number of attempts allowed for the activity	No. of attempts taken by the learner (with date of each attempt)	Any remedial training needed? (Yes / No) If yes then state the reason(s)	Rating 1. Scope for further improvement 2. Satisfactory (All attempts at the activity must be rated separately)	Final decision of faculty C—Completed N—Not completed	Feedback conveyed by faculty (Yes / No) Signature of faculty (with date)	Feedback received by learner (Yes / No) Signature of learner (with date)
61.								
62.								
63.								
64.								
65.								

A. Ist Professional MBBS

Sr. No.	Competency number and description of the activity	Maximum number of attempts allowed for the activity	No. of attempts taken by the learner (with date of each attempt)	Any remedial training needed? (Yes / No) If yes then state the reason(s)	Rating 1. Scope for further improvement 2. Satisfactory (All attempts at the activity must be rated separately)	Final decision of faculty C—Completed N—Not completed	Feedback conveyed by faculty (Yes / No) Signature of faculty (with date)	Feedback received by learner (Yes / No) Signature of learner (with date)
66.								
67.								
68.								
69.								
70.								

B. IInd Professional MBBS

S. No.	Competency number and description of the activity	Maximum number of attempts allowed for the activity	No. of attempts taken by the learner (with date of each attempt)	Any remedial training needed? (Yes / No) If yes then state the reason(s)	Rating 1. Scope for further improvement 2. Satisfactory (All attempts at the activity must be rated separately)	Final decision of faculty C—Completed N—Not completed	Feedback conveyed by faculty (Yes / No) Signature of faculty (with date)	Feedback received by learner (Yes / No) Signature of learner (with date)
1.								
2.								
3.								
4.								
5.								

B. IInd Professional MBBS

Sr. No.	Competency number and description of the activity	Maximum number of attempts allowed for the activity	No. of attempts taken by the learner (with date of each attempt)	Any remedial training needed? (Yes / No) If yes then state the reason(s)	Rating 1. Scope for further improvement 2. Satisfactory (All attempts at the activity must be rated separately)	Final decision of faculty C—Completed N—Not completed	Feedback conveyed by faculty (Yes / No) Signature of faculty (with date)	Feedback received by learner (Yes / No) Signature of learner (with date)
6.								
7.								
8.								
9.								
10.								

B. IInd Professional MBBS

Sr. No.	Competency number and description of the activity	Maximum number of attempts allowed for the activity	No. of attempts taken by the learner (with date of each attempt)	Any remedial training needed? (Yes / No) If yes then state the reason(s)	Rating 1. Scope for further improvement 2. Satisfactory (All attempts at the activity must be rated separately)	Final decision of faculty C—Completed N—Not completed	Feedback conveyed by faculty (Yes / No) Signature of faculty (with date)	Feedback received by learner (Yes / No) Signature of learner (with date)
11.								
12.								
13								
14.								
15.								

B. IInd Professional MBBS

Sr. No.	Competency number and description of the activity	Maximum number of attempts allowed for the activity	No. of attempts taken by the learner (with date of each attempt)	Any remedial training needed? (Yes / No) If yes then state the reason(s)	Rating 1. Scope for further improvement 2. Satisfactory (All attempts at the activity must be rated separately)	Final decision of faculty C—Completed N—Not completed	Feedback conveyed by faculty (Yes / No) Signature of faculty (with date)	Feedback received by learner (Yes / No) Signature of learner (with date)
16.								
17.								
18.								
19.								
20.								

B. IInd Professional MBBS

Sr. No.	Competency number and description of the activity	Maximum number of attempts allowed for the activity	No. of attempts taken by the learner (with date of each attempt)	Any remedial training needed? (Yes / No) If yes then state the reason(s)	Rating 1. Scope for further improvement 2. Satisfactory (All attempts at the activity must be rated separately)	Final decision of faculty C—Completed N—Not completed	Feedback conveyed by faculty (Yes / No) Signature of faculty (with date)	Feedback received by learner (Yes / No) Signature of learner (with date)
21								
22.								
23.								
24.								
25.								

B. IInd Professional MBBS

Sr. No.	Competency number and description of the activity	Maximum number of attempts allowed for the activity	No. of attempts taken by the learner (with date of each attempt)	Any remedial training needed? (Yes / No) If yes then state the reason(s)	Rating 1. Scope for further improvement 2. Satisfactory (All attempts at the activity must be rated separately)	Final decision of faculty C—Completed N—Not completed	Feedback conveyed by faculty (Yes / No) Signature of faculty (with date)	Feedback received by learner (Yes / No) Signature of learner (with date)
26.								
27.								
28.								
29.								
30.								

B. IInd Professional MBBS

Sr. No.	Competency number and description of the activity	Maximum number of attempts allowed for the activity	No. of attempts taken by the learner (with date of each attempt)	Any remedial training needed? (Yes / No) If yes then state the reason(s)	Rating 1. Scope for further improvement 2. Satisfactory (All attempts at the activity must be rated separately)	Final decision of faculty C—Completed N—Not completed	Feedback conveyed by faculty (Yes / No) Signature of faculty (with date)	Feedback received by learner (Yes / No) Signature of learner (with date)
31.								
32.								
33								
34.								
35.								

B. IInd Professional MBBS

Sr. No.	Competency number and description of the activity	Maximum number of attempts allowed for the activity	No. of attempts taken by the learner (with date of each attempt)	Any remedial training needed? (Yes / No) If yes then state the reason(s)	Rating 1. Scope for further improvement 2. Satisfactory (All attempts at the activity must be rated separately)	Final decision of faculty C—Completed N—Not completed	Feedback conveyed by faculty (Yes / No) Signature of faculty (with date)	Feedback received by learner (Yes / No) Signature of learner (with date)
36.								
37.								
38.								
39.								
40.								

B. IInd Professional MBBS

Sr. No.	Competency number and description of the activity	Maximum number of attempts allowed for the activity	No. of attempts taken by the learner (with date of each attempt)	Any remedial training needed? (Yes / No) If yes then state the reason(s)	Rating 1. Scope for further improvement 2. Satisfactory (All attempts at the activity must be rated separately)	Final decision of faculty C—Completed N—Not completed	Feedback conveyed by faculty (Yes / No) Signature of faculty (with date)	Feedback received by learner (Yes / No) Signature of learner (with date)
41.								
42								
43.								
44.								
45.								

B. IInd Professional MBBS

Sr. No.	Competency number and description of the activity	Maximum number of attempts allowed for the activity	No. of attempts taken by the learner (with date of each attempt)	Any remedial training needed? (Yes / No) If yes then state the reason(s)	Rating 1. Scope for further improvement 2. Satisfactory (All attempts at the activity must be rated separately)	Final decision of faculty C—Completed N—Not completed	Feedback conveyed by faculty (Yes / No) Signature of faculty (with date)	Feedback received by learner (Yes / No) Signature of learner (with date)
46.								
47.								
48.								
49.								
50.								

B. IInd Professional MBBS

Sr. No.	Competency number and description of the activity	Maximum number of attempts allowed for the activity	No. of attempts taken by the learner (with date of each attempt)	Any remedial training needed? (Yes / No) If yes then state the reason(s)	Rating 1. Scope for further improvement 2. Satisfactory (All attempts at the activity must be rated separately)	Final decision of faculty C—Completed N—Not completed	Feedback conveyed by faculty (Yes / No) Signature of faculty (with date)	Feedback received by learner (Yes / No) Signature of learner (with date)
51.								
52.								
53.								
54.								
55.								

B. IInd Professional MBBS

Sr. No.	Competency number and description of the activity	Maximum number of attempts allowed for the activity	No. of attempts taken by the learner (with date of each attempt)	Any remedial training needed? (Yes / No) If yes then state the reason(s)	Rating 1. Scope for further improvement 2. Satisfactory (All attempts at the activity must be rated separately)	Final decision of faculty C—Completed N—Not completed	Feedback conveyed by faculty (Yes / No) Signature of faculty (with date)	Feedback received by learner (Yes / No) Signature of learner (with date)
56.								
57.								
58.								
59.								
60.								

B. IInd Professional MBBS

Sr No.	Competency number and description of the activity	Maximum number of attempts allowed for the activity	No. of attempts taken by the learner (with date of each attempt)	Any remedial training needed? (Yes / No) If yes then state the reason(s)	Rating 1. Scope for further improvement 2. Satisfactory (All attempts at the activity must be rated separately)	Final decision of faculty C—Completed N—Not completed	Feedback conveyed by faculty (Yes / No) Signature of faculty (with date)	Feedback received by learner (Yes / No) Signature of learner (with date)
61.								
62.								
63.								
64.								
65.								

B. IInd Professional MBBS

Sr. No.	Competency number and description of the activity	Maximum number of attempts allowed for the activity	No. of attempts taken by the learner (with date of each attempt)	Any remedial training needed? (Yes / No) If yes then state the reason(s)	Rating 1. Scope for further improvement 2. Satisfactory (All attempts at the activity must be rated separately)	Final decision of faculty C—Completed N—Not completed	Feedback conveyed by faculty (Yes / No) Signature of faculty (with date)	Feedback received by learner (Yes / No) Signature of learner (with date)
66.								
67.								
68.								
69.								
70.								

C. IIIrd Professional MBBS (Part I)

Sr. No.	Competency number and description of the activity	Maximum number of attempts allowed for the activity	No. of attempts taken by the learner (with date of each attempt)	Any remedial training needed? (Yes / No) If yes then state the reason(s)	Rating 1. Scope for further improvement 2. Satisfactory (All attempts at the activity must be rated separately)	Final decision of faculty C—Completed N—Not completed	Feedback conveyed by faculty (Yes / No) Signature of faculty (with date)	Feedback received by learner (Yes / No) Signature of learner (with date)
1.								
2.								
3.								
4.								
5.								

C. IIIrd Professional MBBS (Part I)

Sr. No.	Competency number and description of the activity	Maximum number of attempts allowed for the activity	No. of attempts taken by the learner (with date of each attempt)	Any remedial training needed? (Yes / No) If yes then state the reason(s)	Rating 1. Scope for further improvement 2. Satisfactory (All attempts at the activity must be rated separately)	Final decision of faculty C—Completed N—Not completed	Feedback conveyed by faculty (Yes / No) Signature of faculty (with date)	Feedback received by learner (Yes / No) Signature of learner (with date)
6.								
7.								
8.								
9.								
10.								

C. IIIrd Professional MBBS (Part I)

Sr. No.	Competency number and description of the activity	Maximum number of attempts allowed for the activity	No. of attempts taken by the learner (with date of each attempt)	Any remedial training needed? (Yes / No) If yes then state the reason(s)	Rating 1. Scope for further improvement 2. Satisfactory (All attempts at the activity must be rated separately)	Final decision of faculty C—Completed N—Not completed	Feedback conveyed by faculty (Yes / No) Signature of faculty (with date)	Feedback received by learner (Yes / No) Signature of learner (with date)
11.								
12.								
13.								
14.								
15.								

C. IIIrd Professional MBBS (Part I)

Sr. No.	Competency number and description of the activity	Maximum number of attempts allowed for the activity	No. of attempts taken by the learner (with date of each attempt)	Any remedial training needed? (Yes / No) If yes then state the reason(s)	Rating 1. Scope for further improvement 2. Satisfactory (All attempts at the activity must be rated separately)	Final decision of faculty C—Completed N—Not completed	Feedback conveyed by faculty (Yes / No) Signature of faculty (with date)	Feedback received by learner (Yes / No) Signature of learner (with date)
16.								
17.								
18.								
19.								
20.								

C. IIIrd Professional MBBS (Part I)

Sr. No.	Competency number and description of the activity	Maximum number of attempts allowed for the activity	No. of attempts taken by the learner (with date of each attempt)	Any remedial training needed? (Yes / No) If yes then state the reason(s)	Rating 1. Scope for further improvement 2. Satisfactory (All attempts at the activity must be rated separately)	Final decision of faculty C—Completed N—Not completed	Feedback conveyed by faculty (Yes / No) Signature of faculty (with date)	Feedback received by learner (Yes / No) Signature of learner (with date)
21.								
22.								
23.								
24.								
25.								

C. IIIrd Professional MBBS (Part I)

Sr. No.	Competency number and description of the activity	Maximum number of attempts allowed for the activity	No. of attempts taken by the learner (with date of each attempt)	Any remedial training needed? (Yes / No) If yes then state the reason(s)	Rating 1. Scope for further improvement 2. Satisfactory (All attempts at the activity must be rated separately)	Final decision of faculty C—Completed N—Not completed	Feedback conveyed by faculty (Yes / No) Signature of faculty (with date)	Feedback received by learner (Yes / No) Signature of learner (with date)
26.								
27.								
28.								
29.								
30.								

C. IIIrd Professional MBBS (Part I)

Sr. No.	Competency number and description of the activity	Maximum number of attempts allowed for the activity	No. of attempts taken by the learner (with date of each attempt)	Any remedial training needed? (Yes / No) If yes then state the reason(s)	Rating 1. Scope for further improvement 2. Satisfactory (All attempts at the activity must be rated separately)	Final decision of faculty C—Completed N—Not completed	Feedback conveyed by faculty (Yes / No) Signature of faculty (with date)	Feedback received by learner (Yes / No) Signature of learner (with date)
31								
32.								
33.								
34.								
35.								

C. IIIrd Professional MBBS (Part I)

Sr. No.	Competency number and description of the activity	Maximum number of attempts allowed for the activity	No. of attempts taken by the learner (with date of each attempt)	Any remedial training needed? (Yes / No) If yes then state the reason(s)	Rating 1. Scope for further improvement 2. Satisfactory (All attempts at the activity must be rated separately)	Final decision of faculty C—Completed N—Not completed	Feedback conveyed by faculty (Yes / No) Signature of faculty (with date)	Feedback received by learner (Yes / No) Signature of learner (with date)
36.								
37.								
38.								
39.								
40.								

C. IIIrd Professional MBBS (Part I)

Sr. No.	Competency number and description of the activity	Maximum number of attempts allowed for the activity	No. of attempts taken by the learner (with date of each attempt)	Any remedial training needed? (Yes / No) If yes then state the reason(s)	Rating 1. Scope for further improvement 2. Satisfactory (All attempts at the activity must be rated separately)	Final decision of faculty C—Completed N—Not completed	Feedback conveyed by faculty (Yes / No) Signature of faculty (with date)	Feedback received by learner (Yes / No) Signature of learner (with date)
41.								
42.								
43								
44.								
45.								

C. IIIrd Professional MBBS (Part I)

Sr. No.	Competency number and description of the activity	Maximum number of attempts allowed for the activity	No. of attempts taken by the learner (with date of each attempt)	Any remedial training needed? (Yes / No) If yes then state the reason(s)	Rating 1. Scope for further improvement 2. Satisfactory (All attempts at the activity must be rated separately)	Final decision of faculty C—Completed N—Not completed	Feedback conveyed by faculty (Yes / No) Signature of faculty (with date)	Feedback received by learner (Yes / No) Signature of learner (with date)
46.								
47.								
48.								
49.								
50.								

C. IIIrd Professional MBBS (Part I)

Sr. No.	Competency number and description of the activity	Maximum number of attempts allowed for the activity	No. of attempts taken by the learner (with date of each attempt)	Any remedial training needed? (Yes / No) If yes then state the reason(s)	Rating 1. Scope for further improvement 2. Satisfactory (All attempts at the activity must be rated separately)	Final decision of faculty C—Completed N—Not completed	Feedback conveyed by faculty (Yes / No) Signature of faculty (with date)	Feedback received by learner (Yes / No) Signature of learner (with date)
51.								
52.								
53								
54.								
55.								

C. IIIrd Professional MBBS (Part I)

Sr. No.	Competency number and description of the activity	Maximum number of attempts allowed for the activity	No. of attempts taken by the learner (with date of each attempt)	Any remedial training needed? (Yes / No) If yes then state the reason(s)	Rating 1. Scope for further improvement 2. Satisfactory (All attempts at the activity must be rated separately)	Final decision of faculty C—Completed N—Not completed	Feedback conveyed by faculty (Yes / No) Signature of faculty (with date)	Feedback received by learner (Yes / No) Signature of learner (with date)
56.								
57.								
58.								
59.								
60.								

C. IIIrd Professional MBBS (Part I)

S. No.	Competency number and description of the activity	Maximum number of attempts allowed for the activity	No. of attempts taken by the learner (with date of each attempt)	Any remedial training needed? (Yes / No) If yes then state the reason(s)	Rating 1. Scope for further improvement 2. Satisfactory (All attempts at the activity must be rated separately)	Final decision of faculty C—Completed N—Not completed	Feedback conveyed by faculty (Yes / No) Signature of faculty (with date)	Feedback received by learner (Yes / No) Signature of learner (with date)
61.								
62.								
63.								
64.								
65.								

C. IIIrd Professional MBBS (Part I)

Sr. No.	Competency number and description of the activity	Maximum number of attempts allowed for the activity	No. of attempts taken by the learner (with date of each attempt)	Any remedial training needed? (Yes / No) If yes then state the reason(s)	Rating 1. Scope for further improvement 2. Satisfactory (All attempts at the activity must be rated separately)	Final decision of faculty C—Completed N—Not completed	Feedback conveyed by faculty (Yes / No) Signature of faculty (with date)	Feedback received by learner (Yes / No) Signature of learner (with date)
66.								
67.								
68.								
69.								
70.								

D. IIIrd Professional MBBS (Part II)

Sr. No.	Competency number and description of the activity	Maximum number of attempts allowed for the activity	No. of attempts taken by the learner (with date of each attempt)	Any remedial training needed? (Yes / No) If yes then state the reason(s)	Rating 1. Scope for further improvement 2. Satisfactory (All attempts at the activity must be rated separately)	Final decision of faculty C—Completed N—Not completed	Feedback conveyed by faculty (Yes / No) Signature of faculty (with date)	Feedback received by learner (Yes / No) Signature of learner (with date)
1.								
2.								
3.								
4.								
5.								

D. IIIrd Professional MBBS (Part II)

Sr. No.	Competency number and description of the activity	Maximum number of attempts allowed for the activity	No. of attempts taken by the learner (with date of each attempt)	Any remedial training needed? (Yes / No) If yes then state the reason(s)	Rating 1. Scope for further improvement 2. Satisfactory (All attempts at the activity must be rated separately)	Final decision of faculty C—Completed N—Not completed	Feedback conveyed by faculty (Yes / No) Signature of faculty (with date)	Feedback received by learner (Yes / No) Signature of learner (with date)
6.								
7.								
8.								
9.								
10.								

D. IIIrd Professional MBBS (Part II)

Sr. No.	Competency number and description of the activity	Maximum number of attempts allowed for the activity	No. of attempts taken by the learner (with date of each attempt)	Any remedial training needed? (Yes / No) If yes then state the reason(s)	Rating 1. Scope for further improvement 2. Satisfactory (All attempts at the activity must be rated separately)	Final decision of faculty C—Completed N—Not completed	Feedback conveyed by faculty (Yes / No) Signature of faculty (with date)	Feedback received by learner (Yes / No) Signature of learner (with date)
11.								
12.								
13.								
14.								
15.								

D. IIIrd Professional MBBS (Part II)

Sr. No.	Competency number and description of the activity	Maximum number of attempts allowed for the activity	No. of attempts taken by the learner (with date of each attempt)	Any remedial training needed? (Yes / No) If yes then state the reason(s)	Rating 1. Scope for further improvement 2. Satisfactory (All attempts at the activity must be rated separately)	Final decision of faculty C—Completed N—Not completed	Feedback conveyed by faculty (Yes / No) Signature of faculty (with date)	Feedback received by learner (Yes / No) Signature of learner (with date)
16.								
17.								
18.								
19.								
20.								

D. IIIrd Professional MBBS (Part II)

Sr. No.	Competency number and description of the activity	Maximum number of attempts allowed for the activity	No. of attempts taken by the learner (with date of each attempt)	Any remedial training needed? (Yes / No) If yes then state the reason(s)	Rating 1. Scope for further improvement 2. Satisfactory (All attempts at the activity must be rated separately)	Final decision of faculty C—Completed N—Not completed	Feedback conveyed by faculty (Yes / No) Signature of faculty (with date)	Feedback received by learner (Yes / No) Signature of learner (with date)
21.								
22.								
23.								
24.								
25.								

D. IIIrd Professional MBBS (Part II)

Sr. No.	Competency number and description of the activity	Maximum number of attempts allowed for the activity	No. of attempts taken by the learner (with date of each attempt)	Any remedial training needed? (Yes / No) If yes then state the reason(s)	Rating 1. Scope for further improvement 2. Satisfactory (All attempts at the activity must be rated separately)	Final decision of faculty C—Completed N—Not completed	Feedback conveyed by faculty (Yes / No) Signature of faculty (with date)	Feedback received by learner (Yes / No) Signature of learner (with date)
26.								
27.								
28.								
29.								
30.								

D. IIIrd Professional MBBS (Part II)

Sr. No.	Competency number and description of the activity	Maximum number of attempts allowed for the activity	No. of attempts taken by the learner (with date of each attempt)	Any remedial training needed? (Yes / No) If yes then state the reason(s)	Rating 1. Scope for further improvement 2. Satisfactory (All attempts at the activity must be rated separately)	Final decision of faculty C—Completed N—Not completed	Feedback conveyed by faculty (Yes / No) Signature of faculty (with date)	Feedback received by learner (Yes / No) Signature of learner (with date)
31.								
32.								
33.								
34.								
35.								

D. IIIrd Professional MBBS (Part II)

Sr. No.	Competency number and description of the activity	Maximum number of attempts allowed for the activity	No. of attempts taken by the learner (with date of each attempt)	Any remedial training needed? (Yes / No) If yes then state the reason(s)	Rating 1. Scope for further improvement 2. Satisfactory (All attempts at the activity must be rated separately)	Final decision of faculty C—Completed N—Not completed	Feedback conveyed by faculty (Yes / No) Signature of faculty (with date)	Feedback received by learner (Yes / No) Signature of learner (with date)
36.								
37.								
38.								
39.								
40.								

D. IIIrd Professional MBBS (Part II)

Sr. No.	Competency number and description of the activity	Maximum number of attempts allowed for the activity	No. of attempts taken by the learner (with date of each attempt)	Any remedial training needed? (Yes / No) If yes then state the reason(s)	Rating 1. Scope for further improvement 2. Satisfactory (All attempts at the activity must be rated separately)	Final decision of faculty C—Completed N—Not completed	Feedback conveyed by faculty (Yes / No) Signature of faculty (with date)	Feedback received by learner (Yes / No) Signature of learner (with date)
41.								
42.								
43.								
44.								
45.								

D. IIIrd Professional MBBS (Part II)

Sr. No.	Competency number and description of the activity	Maximum number of attempts allowed for the activity	No. of attempts taken by the learner (with date of each attempt)	Any remedial training needed? (Yes / No) If yes then state the reason(s)	Rating 1. Scope for further improvement 2. Satisfactory (All attempts at the activity must be rated separately)	Final decision of faculty C—Completed N—Not completed	Feedback conveyed by faculty (Yes / No) Signature of faculty (with date)	Feedback received by learner (Yes / No) Signature of learner (with date)
46.								
47.								
48.								
49.								
50.								

D. IIIrd Professional MBBS (Part II)

Sr. No.	Competency number and description of the activity	Maximum number of attempts allowed for the activity	No. of attempts taken by the learner (with date of each attempt)	Any remedial training needed? (Yes / No) If yes then state the reason(s)	Rating 1. Scope for further improvement 2. Satisfactory (All attempts at the activity must be rated separately)	Final decision of faculty C—Completed N—Not completed	Feedback conveyed by faculty (Yes / No) Signature of faculty (with date)	Feedback received by learner (Yes / No) Signature of learner (with date)
51.								
52.								
53.								
54.								
55.								

D. IIIrd Professional MBBS (Part II)

Sr. No.	Competency number and description of the activity	Maximum number of attempts allowed for the activity	No. of attempts taken by the learner (with date of each attempt)	Any remedial training needed? (Yes / No) If yes then state the reason(s)	Rating 1. Scope for further improvement 2. Satisfactory (All attempts at the activity must be rated separately)	Final decision of faculty C—Completed N—Not completed	Feedback conveyed by faculty (Yes / No) Signature of faculty (with date)	Feedback received by learner (Yes / No) Signature of learner (with date)
56.								
57.								
58.								
59.								
60.								

D. IIIrd Professional MBBS (Part II)

Sr. No.	Competency number and description of the activity	Maximum number of attempts allowed for the activity	No. of attempts taken by the learner (with date of each attempt)	Any remedial training needed? (Yes / No) If yes then state the reason(s)	Rating 1. Scope for further improvement 2. Satisfactory (All attempts at the activity must be rated separately)	Final decision of faculty C—Completed N—Not completed	Feedback conveyed by faculty (Yes / No) Signature of faculty (with date)	Feedback received by learner (Yes / No) Signature of learner (with date)
61.								
62.								
63.								
64.								
65								

D. IIIrd Professional MBBS (Part II)

Sr. No.	Competency number and description of the activity	Maximum number of attempts allowed for the activity	No. of attempts taken by the learner (with date of each attempt)	Any remedial training needed? (Yes / No) If yes then state the reason(s)	Rating 1. Scope for further improvement 2. Satisfactory (All attempts at the activity must be rated separately)	Final decision of faculty C—Completed N—Not completed	Feedback conveyed by faculty (Yes / No) Signature of faculty (with date)	Feedback received by learner (Yes / No) Signature of learner (with date)
66.								
67.								
68.								
69.								
70.								

Section 2

Medical Humanities

Medical Humanities

The Centre for Medical Humanities, Royal Free and University College Medical School, London, England defines Medical Humanities as

'*An interdisciplinary, and increasingly international endeavour that draws on the creative and intellectual strengths of diverse disciplines, including literature, art, creative writing, drama, film, music, philosophy, ethical decision making, anthropology, and history, in pursuit of medical educational goals.'*

Medical Humanities is being formally introduced under the new Competency Based Medical Education (CBME) curriculum. It is a revolutionary way of thinking and viewing everything around us with a different (and unique) perspective.

Medical Humanities goes one step beyond communication skills or knowledge of medical ethics; it allows us to appreciate the individuality of human beings and can help healthcare professionals in dealing with ethical dilemmas and difficult decision making. We hope that by attending these sessions the learners will understand and appreciate the 'human' side of medicine.

*Reference

Kirklin, Deborah BM, BCh, MA, MRCGP. The Centre for Medical Humanities, Royal Free and University College Medical School, London, England, Academic Medicine: October 2003; Volume 78; Issue 10; p 1048–53.

Reflective Portfolio

A. lst Professional MBBS

Session details	Please describe briefly what happened during the session	What did you learn from the session?	Do you feel that the knowledge you have acquired in this session will help you become a better doctor? Please explain in your own words.
Session 1 Name of the session Name of faculty member(s) Date Time Duration			
Session 2 Name of the session Name of faculty member(s) Date Time Duration			
Session 3 Name of the session Name of faculty member(s) Date Time Duration			
Session 4 Name of the session Name of faculty member(s) Date Time Duration			

Reflective Portfolio

A. Ist Professional MBBS

Session details	Please describe briefly what happened during the session	What did you learn from the session?	Do you feel that the knowledge you have acquired in this session will help you become a better doctor? Please explain in your own words.
Session 5 Name of the session Name of faculty member(s) Date Time Duration			
Session 6 Name of the session Name of faculty member(s) Date Time Duration			
Session 7 Name of the session Name of faculty member(s) Date Time Duration			
Session 8 Name of the session Name of faculty member(s) Date Time Duration			

Reflective Portfolio

A. Ist Professional MBBS

Session details	Please describe briefly what happened during the session	What did you learn from the session?	Do you feel that the knowledge you have acquired in this session will help you become a better doctor? Please explain in your own words.
Session 9 Name of the session Name of faculty member(s) Date Time Duration			
Session 10 Name of the session Name of faculty member(s) Date Time Duration			
Session 11 Name of the session Name of faculty member(s) Date Time Duration			
Session 12 Name of the session Name of faculty member(s) Date Time Duration			

Reflective Portfolio

A. Ist Professional MBBS

Session details	Please describe briefly what happened during the session	What did you learn from the session?	Do you feel that the knowledge you have acquired in this session will help you become a better doctor? Please explain in your own words.
Session 13 Name of the session Name of faculty member(s) Date Time Duration			
Session 14 Name of the session Name of faculty member(s) Date Time Duration			
Session 15 Name of the session Name of faculty member(s) Date Time Duration			
Session 16 Name of the session Name of faculty member(s) Date Time Duration			

Reflective Portfolio

A. Ist Professional MBBS

Session details	Please describe briefly what happened during the session	What did you learn from the session?	Do you feel that the knowledge you have acquired in this session will help you become a better doctor? Please explain in your own words.
Session 17 Name of the session Name of faculty member(s) Date Time Duration			
Session 18 Name of the session Name of faculty member(s) Date Time Duration			
Session 19 Name of the session Name of faculty member(s) Date Time Duration			
Session 20 Name of the session Name of faculty member(s) Date Time Duration			

Reflective Portfolio

A. Ist Professional MBBS

Session details	Please describe briefly what happened during the session	What did you learn from the session?	Do you feel that the knowledge you have acquired in this session will help you become a better doctor? Please explain in your own words.
Session 21 Name of the session Name of faculty member(s) Date Time Duration			
Session 22 Name of the session Name of faculty member(s) Date Time Duration			
Session 23 Name of the session Name of faculty member(s) Date Time Duration			
Session 24 Name of the session Name of faculty member(s) Date Time Duration			

Reflective Portfolio

A. Ist Professional MBBS

Session details	Please describe briefly what happened during the session	What did you learn from the session?	Do you feel that the knowledge you have acquired in this session will help you become a better doctor? Please explain in your own words.
Session 25 Name of the session Name of faculty member(s) Date Time Duration			
Session 26 Name of the session Name of faculty member(s) Date Time Duration			
Session 27 Name of the session Name of faculty member(s) Date Time Duration			
Session 28 Name of the session Name of faculty member(s) Date Time Duration			

Details of Assignments and Assessments

Please record any assignments and/or assessments on this page.

Suggested Format
a. Topic
b. Date
c. Details of assignment/assessment
d. Feedback received (Yes/No)
e. Reflection writing

Details of Assignments and Assessments

Please record any assignments and/or assessments on this page.

Suggested Format
a. Topic
b. Date
c. Details of assignment/assessment
d. Feedback received (Yes/No)
e. Reflection writing

Details of Assignments and Assessments

Please record any assignments and/or assessments on this page.

Suggested Format

a. Topic

b. Date

c. Details of assignment/assessment

d. Feedback received (Yes/No)

e. Reflection writing

Details of Assignments and Assessments

Please record any assignments and/or assessments on this page.

Suggested Format
a. Topic
b. Date
c. Details of assignment/assessment
d. Feedback received (Yes/No)
e. Reflection writing

Reflective Portfolio

B. IInd Professional MBBS

Session details	Please describe briefly what happened during the session	What did you learn from the session?	Do you feel that the knowledge you have acquired in this session will help you become a better doctor? Please explain in your own words.
Session 1 Name of the session Name of faculty member(s) Date Time Duration			
Session 2 Name of the session Name of faculty member(s) Date Time Duration			
Session 3 Name of the session Name of faculty member(s) Date Time Duration			
Session 4 Name of the session Name of faculty member(s) Date Time Duration			

Reflective Portfolio
B. IInd Professional MBBS

Session details	Please describe briefly what happened during the session	What did you learn from the session?	Do you feel that the knowledge you have acquired in this session will help you become a better doctor? Please explain in your own words.
Session 5 Name of the session Name of faculty member(s) Date Time Duration			
Session 6 Name of the session Name of faculty member(s) Date Time Duration			
Session 7 Name of the session Name of faculty member(s) Date Time Duration			
Sess on 8 Name of the session Name of faculty member(s) Date Time Duraton			

Reflective Portfolio

B. IInd Professional MBBS

Session details	Please describe briefly what happened during the session	What did you learn from the session?	Do you feel that the knowledge you have acquired in this session will help you become a better doctor? Please explain in your own words.
Session 9 Name of the session Name of faculty member(s) Date Time Duration			
Session 10 Name of the session Name of faculty member(s) Date Time Duration			
Session 11 Name of the session Name of faculty member(s) Date Time Duration			
Session 12 Name of the session Name of faculty member(s) Date Time Duration			

Details of Assignments and Assessments

Please record any assignments and/or assessments on this page.

Suggested Format
a. Topic
b. Date
c. Details of assignment/assessment
d. Feedback received (Yes/No)
e. Reflection writing

Details of Assignments and Assessments

Please record any assignments and/or assessments on this page.

Suggested Format
a. Topic
b. Date
c. Details of assignment/assessment
d. Feedback received (Yes/No)
e. Reflection writing

Reflective Portfolio
C. IIIrd Professional MBBS (Part I)

Session details	Please describe briefly what happened during the session	What did you learn from the session?	Do you feel that the knowledge you have acquired in this session will help you become a better doctor? Please explain in your own words.
Sess on 1 Name of the session Name of faculty member(s) Date Time Durat on			
Session 2 Name of the session Name of faculty member(s) Date Time Durat on			
Session 3 Name of the session Name of faculty member(s) Date Time Durat on			
Session 4 Name of the session Name of faculty member(s) Date Time Durat on			

Reflective Portfolio
C. IIIrd Professional MBBS (Part I)

Session details	Please describe briefly what happened during the session	What did you learn from the session?	Do you feel that the knowledge you have acquired in this session will help you become a better doctor? Please explain in your own words.
Session 5 Name of the session Name of faculty member(s) Date Time Duration			
Session 6 Name of the session Name of faculty member(s) Date Time Duration			
Session 7 Name of the session Name of faculty member(s) Date Time Duration			
Session 8 Name of the session Name of faculty member(s) Date Time Duration			

Reflective Portfolio
C. IIIrd Professional MBBS (Part I)

Session details	Please describe briefly what happened during the session	What did you learn from the session?	Do you feel that the knowledge you have acquired in this session will help you become a better doctor? Please explain in your own words.
Session 9 Name of the session Name of faculty member(s) Date Time Duration			
Session 10 Name of the session Name of faculty member(s) Date Time Duration			
Session 11 Name of the session Name of faculty member(s) Date Time Duration			
Session 12 Name of the session Name of faculty member(s) Date Time Duration			

Details of Assignments and Assessments

Please record any assignments and/or assessments on this page.

Suggested Format
a. Topic
b. Date
c. Details of assignment/assessment
d. Feedback received (Yes/No)
e. Reflection writing

Details of Assignments and Assessments

Please record any assignments and/or assessments on this page.

Suggested Format
a. Topic
b. Date
c. Details of assignment/assessment
d. Feedback received (Yes/No)
e. Reflection writing

Reflective Portfolio
D. IIIrd Professional MBBS (Part II)

Session details	Please describe briefly what happened during the session	What did you learn from the session?	Do you feel that the knowledge you have acquired in this session will help you become a better doctor? Please explain in your own words.
Session 1 Name of the session Name of faculty member(s) Date Time Duration			
Session 2 Name of the session Name of faculty member(s) Date Time Duration			
Session 3 Name of the session Name of faculty member(s) Date Time Duration			
Session 4 Name of the session Name of faculty member(s) Date Time Duration			

Reflective Portfolio
D. IIIrd Professional MBBS (Part II)

Session details	Please describe briefly what happened during the session	What did you learn from the session?	Do you feel that the knowledge you have acquired in this session will help you become a better doctor? Please explain in your own words.
Session 5 Name of the session Name of faculty member(s) Date Time Duration			
Session 6 Name of the session Name of faculty member(s) Date Time Duration			
Session 7 Name of the session Name of faculty member(s) Date Time Duration			
Session 8 Name of the session Name of faculty member(s) Date Time Duration			

Reflective Portfolio

D. IIIrd Professional MBBS (Part II)

Session details	Please describe briefly what happened during the session	What did you learn from the session?	Do you feel that the knowledge you have acquired in this session will help you become a better doctor? Please explain in your own words.
Session 9 Name of the session Name of faculty member(s) Date Time Duration			
Session 10 Name of the session Name of faculty member(s) Date Time Duration			
Session 11 Name of the session Name of faculty member(s) Date Time Duration			
Session 12 Name of the session Name of faculty member(s) Date Time Duration			

Details of Assignments and Assessments

Please record any assignments and/or assessments on this page.

Suggested Format
a. Topic
b. Date
c. Details of assignment/assessment
d. Feedback received (Yes/No)
e. Reflection writing

Details of Assignments and Assessments

Please record any assignments and/or assessments on this page.

Suggested Format

a. Topic
b. Date
c. Details of assignment/assessment
d. Feedback received (Yes/No)
e. Reflection writing

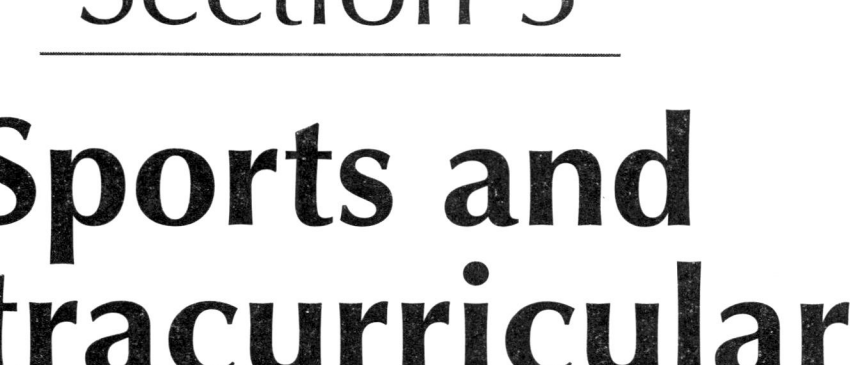

Section 3

Sports and Extracurricular Activities

Reflective Portfolio
A. Ist Professional MBBS

Session details	Please describe briefly what happened during the session	What did you learn from the session?	Do you feel that the knowledge you have acquired in this session will help you become a better doctor? Please explain in your own words.
Session 1 Name of the session Name of faculty member(s) Date Time Duration			
Session 2 Name of the session Name of faculty member(s) Date Time Duration			
Session 3 Name of the session Name of faculty member(s) Date Time Duration			
Session 4 Name of the session Name of faculty member(s) Date Time Duration			

Reflective Portfolio

A. Ist Professional MBBS

Session details	Please describe briefly what happened during the session	What did you learn from the session?	Do you feel that the knowledge you have acquired in this session will help you become a better doctor? Please explain in your own words.
Session 5 Name of the session Name of faculty member(s) Date Time Duration			
Session 6 Name of the session Name of faculty member(s) Date Time Duration			
Session 7 Name of the session Name of faculty member(s) Date Time Duration			
Session 8 Name of the session Name of faculty member(s) Date Time Duration			

Reflective Portfolio
A. Ist Professional MBBS

Session details	Please describe briefly what happened during the session	What did you learn from the session?	Do you feel that the knowledge you have acquired in this session will help you become a better doctor? Please explain in your own words.
Session 9 Name of the session Name of faculty member(s) Date Time Duration			
Session 10 Name of the session Name of faculty member(s) Date Time Duration			
Session 11 Name of the session Name of faculty member(s) Date Time Duration			
Session 12 Name of the session Name of faculty member(s) Date Time Duration			

Reflective Portfolio

A. Ist Professional MBBS

Session details	Please describe briefly what happened during the session	What did you learn from the session?	Do you feel that the knowledge you have acquired in this session will help you become a better doctor? Please explain in your own words.
Session 13 Name of the session Name of faculty member(s) Date Time Duration			
Session 14 Name of the session Name of faculty member(s) Date Time Duration			
Session 15 Name of the session Name of faculty member(s) Date Time Duration			
Session 16 Name of the session Name of faculty member(s) Date Time Duration			

Reflective Portfolio

A. Ist Professional MBBS

Session details	Please describe briefly what happened during the session	What did you learn from the session?	Do you feel that the knowledge you have acquired in this session will help you become a better doctor? Please explain in your own words.
Session 17 Name of the session Name of faculty member(s) Date Time Duration			
Session 18 Name of the session Name of faculty member(s) Date Time Duration			
Session 19 Name of the session Name of faculty member(s) Date Time Duration			
Session 20 Name of the session Name of faculty member(s) Date Time Duration			

Reflective Portfolio
A. Ist Professional MBBS

Session details	Please describe briefly what happened during the session	What did you learn from the session?	Do you feel that the knowledge you have acquired in this session will help you become a better doctor? Please explain in your own words.
Session 21 Name of the session Name of faculty member(s) Date Time Duration			
Session 22 Name of the session Name of faculty member(s) Date Time Duration			
Session 23 Name of the session Name of faculty member(s) Date Time Duration			
Session 24 Name of the session Name of faculty member(s) Date Time Duration			

Reflective Portfolio

A. Ist Professional MBBS

Session details	Please describe briefly what happened during the session	What did you learn from the session?	Do you feel that the knowledge you have acquired in this session will help you become a better doctor? Please explain in your own words.
Session 25 Name of the session Name of faculty member(s) Date Time Duration			
Session 26 Name of the session Name of faculty member(s) Date Time Duration			
Session 27 Name of the session Name of faculty member(s) Date Time Duration			
Session 28 Name of the session Name of faculty member(s) Date Time Duration			

Reflective Portfolio

A. Ist Professional MBBS

Session details	Please describe briefly what happened during the session	What did you learn from the session?	Do you feel that the knowledge you have acquired in this session will help you become a better doctor? Please explain in your own words.
Session 29 Name of the session Name of faculty member(s) Date Time Duration			
Session 30 Name of the session Name of faculty member(s) Date Time Duration			
Session 31 Name of the session Name of faculty member(s) Date Time Duration			
Session 32 Name of the session Name of faculty member(s) Date Time Duration			

Reflective Portfolio

A. Ist Professional MBBS

Session details	Please describe briefly what happened during the session	What did you learn from the session?	Do you feel that the knowledge you have acquired in this session will help you become a better doctor? Please explain in your own words.
Session 33 Name of the session Name of faculty member(s) Date Time Duration			
Session 34 Name of the session Name of faculty member(s) Date Time Duration			
Session 35 Name of the session Name of faculty member(s) Date Time Duration			
Session 36 Name of the session Name of faculty member(s) Date Time Duration			

Reflective Portfolio

A. Ist Professional MBBS

Session details	Please describe briefly what happened during the session	What did you learn from the session?	Do you feel that the knowledge you have acquired in this session will help you become a better doctor? Please explain in your own words.
Session 37 Name of the session Name of faculty member(s) Date Time Duration			
Session 38 Name of the session Name of faculty member(s) Date Time Duration			
Session 39 Name of the session Name of faculty member(s) Date Time Duration			
Session 40 Name of the session Name of faculty member(s) Date Time Duration			

Reflective Portfolio

A. Ist Professional MBBS

Session details	Please describe briefly what happened during the session	What did you learn from the session?	Do you feel that the knowledge you have acquired in this session will help you become a better doctor? Please explain in your own words.
Session 41 Name of the session Name of faculty member(s) Date Time Duration			
Session 42 Name of the session Name of faculty member(s) Date Time Duration			
Session 43 Name of the session Name of faculty member(s) Date Time Duration			
Session 44 Name of the session Name of faculty member(s) Date Time Duration			

Reflective Portfolio

A. Ist Professional MBBS

Session details	Please describe briefly what happened during the session	What did you learn from the session?	Do you feel that the knowledge you have acquired in this session will help you become a better doctor? Please explain in your own words.
Session 45 Name of the session Name of faculty member(s) Date Time Duration			
Session 46 Name of the session Name of faculty member(s) Date Time Duration			
Session 47 Name of the session Name of faculty member(s) Date Time Duration			
Session 48 Name of the session Name of faculty member(s) Date Time Duration			

Reflective Portfolio

A. Ist Professional MBBS

Session details	Please describe briefly what happened during the session	What did you learn from the session?	Do you feel that the knowledge you have acquired in this session will help you become a better doctor? Please explain in your own words.
Session 49 Name of the session Name of faculty member(s) Date Time Duration			
Sess on 50 Name of the session Name of faculty member(s) Date Time Duration			
Sess on 51 Name of the session Name of faculty member(s) Date Time Duration			
Sess on 52 Name of the session Name of faculty member(s) Date Time Duration			

Reflective Portfolio

A. Ist Professional MBBS

Session details	Please describe briefly what happened during the session	What did you learn from the session?	Do you feel that the knowledge you have acquired in this session will help you become a better doctor? Please explain in your own words.
Session 53 Name of the session Name of faculty member(s) Date Time Duration			
Session 54 Name of the session Name of faculty member(s) Date Time Duration			
Session 55 Name of the session Name of faculty member(s) Date Time Duration			
Session 56 Name of the session Name of faculty member(s) Date Time Duration			

Reflective Portfolio

A. Ist Professional MBBS

Session details	Please describe briefly what happened during the session	What did you learn from the session?	Do you feel that the knowledge you have acquired in this session will help you become a better doctor? Please explain in your own words.
Session 57 Name of the session Name of faculty member(s) Date Time Duration			
Session 58 Name of the session Name of faculty member(s) Date Time Duration			
Session 59 Name of the session Name of faculty member(s) Date Time Duration			
Session 60 Name of the session Name of faculty member(s) Date Time Duration			

Details of Assignments and Assessments

Please record any assignments and/or assessments on this page.

Suggested Format
a. Topic
b. Date
c. Details of assignment/assessment
d. Feedback received (Yes/No)
e. Reflection writing

Details of Assignments and Assessments

Please record any assignments and/or assessments on this page.

Suggested Format
a. Topic
b. Date
c. Details of assignment/assessment
d. Feedback received (Yes/No)
e. Reflection writing

Details of Assignments and Assessments

Please record any assignments and/or assessments on this page.

Suggested Format

a. Topic
b. Date
c. Details of assignment/assessment
d. Feedback received (Yes/No)
e. Reflection writing

Details of Assignments and Assessments

Please record any assignments and/or assessments on this page.

Suggested Format
a. Topic
b. Date
c. Details of assignment/assessment
d. Feedback received (Yes/No)
e. Reflection writing

Reflective Portfolio

B. IInd Professional MBBS

Session details	Please describe briefly what happened during the session	What did you learn from the session?	Do you feel that the knowledge you have acquired in this session will help you become a better doctor? Please explain in your own words.
Session 1 Name of the session Name of faculty member(s) Date Time Duration			
Session 2 Name of the session Name of faculty member(s) Date Time Duration			
Session 3 Name of the session Name of faculty member(s) Date Time Duration			
Session 4 Name of the session Name of faculty member(s) Date Time Duration			

Reflective Portfolio
B. IInd Professional MBBS

Session details	Please describe briefly what happened during the session	What did you learn from the session?	Do you feel that the knowledge you have acquired in this session will help you become a better doctor? Please explain in your own words.
Session 5 Name of the session Name of faculty member(s) Date Time Duration			
Session 6 Name of the session Name of faculty member(s) Date Time Duration			
Session 7 Name of the session Name of faculty member(s) Date Time Duration			
Session 8 Name of the session Name of faculty member(s) Date Time Duration			

Reflective Portfolio
B. IInd Professional MBBS

Session details	Please describe briefly what happened during the session	What did you learn from the session?	Do you feel that the knowledge you have acquired in this session will help you become a better doctor? Please explain in your own words.
Session 9 Name of the session Name of faculty member(s) Date Time Duration			
Session 10 Name of the session Name of faculty member(s) Date Time Duration			
Session 11 Name of the session Name of faculty member(s) Date Time Duration			
Session 12 Name of the session Name of faculty member(s) Date Time Duration			

Reflective Portfolio
B. IInd Professional MBBS

Session details	Please describe briefly what happened during the session	What did you learn from the session?	Do you feel that the knowledge you have acquired in this session will help you become a better doctor? Please explain in your own words.
Session 13 Name of the session Name of faculty member(s) Date Time Duration			
Session 14 Name of the session Name of faculty member(s) Date Time Duration			
Session 15 Name of the session Name of faculty member(s) Date Time Duration			
Session 16 Name of the session Name of faculty member(s) Date Time Duration			

Reflective Portfolio
B. IInd Professional MBBS

Session details	Please describe briefly what happened during the session	What did you learn from the session?	Do you feel that the knowledge you have acquired in this session will help you become a better doctor? Please explain in your own words.
Session 17 Name of the session Name of faculty member(s) Date Time Duration			
Session 18 Name of the session Name of faculty member(s) Date Time Duration			
Session 19 Name of the session Name of faculty member(s) Date Time Duration			
Session 20 Name of the session Name of faculty member(s) Date Time Duration			

Reflective Portfolio
B. IInd Professional MBBS

Session details	Please describe briefly what happened during the session	What did you learn from the session?	Do you feel that the knowledge you have acquired in this session will help you become a better doctor? Please explain in your own words.
Session 21 Name of the session Name of faculty member(s) Date Time Duration			
Session 22 Name of the session Name of faculty member(s) Date Time Duration			
Session 23 Name of the session Name of faculty member(s) Date Time Duration			
Session 24 Name of the session Name of faculty member(s) Date Time Duration			

Reflective Portfolio

B. IInd Professional MBBS

Session details	Please describe briefly what happened during the session	What did you learn from the session?	Do you feel that the knowledge you have acquired in this session will help you become a better doctor? Please explain in your own words.
Session 25 Name of the session Name of faculty member(s) Date Time Duration			
Session 26 Name of the session Name of faculty member(s) Date Time Duration			
Session 27 Name of the session Name of faculty member(s) Date Time Duration			
Session 28 Name of the session Name of faculty member(s) Date Time Duration			

Details of Assignments and Assessments

Please record any assignments and/or assessments on this page.

Suggested Format
a. Topic
b. Date
c. Details of assignment/assessment
d. Feedback received (Yes/No)
e. Reflection writing

Details of Assignments and Assessments

Please record any assignments and/or assessments on this page.

Suggested Format
a. Topic
b. Date
c. Details of assignment/assessment
d. Feedback received (Yes/No)
e. Reflection writing

Details of Assignments and Assessments

Please record any assignments and/or assessments on this page.

Suggested Format
a. Topic
b. Date
c. Details of assignment/assessment
d. Feedback received (Yes/No)
e. Reflection writing

Details of Assignments and Assessments

Please record any assignments and/or assessments on this page.

Suggested Format
a. Topic
b. Date
c. Details of assignment/assessment
d. Feedback received (Yes/No)
e. Reflection writing

FINAL SUMMARY

Sr. No.	Section	Dates (dd/mm/yy)	Overall Assessment (Complete / Incomplete)	Signature of the Faculty-in-charge / HoD (with date)
Ist Professional MBBS				
I.	Attitude, Ethics and Communication (AETCOM)			
2.	Medical Humanities			
3.	Sports and Extracurricular Activities			
IInd Professional MBBS				
1.	Attitude, Ethics and Communication (AETCOM)			
2.	Medical Humanities			
3.	Sports and Extracurricular Activities			
IIIrd Professional MBBS (Part I)				
1.	Attitude, Ethics and Communication (AETCOM)			
2.	Medical Humanities			
IIIrd Professional MBBS (Part II)				
1.	Attitude, Ethics and Communication (AETCOM)			
2.	Medical Humanities			